# Human Sexuality in
# St. John Paul II and Teilhard de Chardin

Bernard J. Fleury, Ed.D.

Human Sexuality                                                    Bernard J. Fleury Ed.D.

*Printed by Create Space, an Amazon.com Company.*

*ISBN-13: 978-1544761565*

*ISBN-10: 1544761562*

*Website:* www.intolifebylight.com

*Printed in the United States of America*

## Table of Contents

Author Biography: Meet Bernard Video and Narrative. www.intolifebylight.com/about/author

LinkedIn Profile: www.linkedin.com/in/bernard-fleury-a4411541

## Description

### Article 1 and the entire e-Book:

Know that man, made in the image and likeness of God is a person created for his own sake, not an animal created as a thing to be used by others.

### Article 2:

What if the human is unique among God's creation?

### Article 3:

What if among all living animal bodies, the human body is unique?

### Article 4:

What if our bodies, male and female, reveal who we are scientifically and theologically?

What if couples living together before marriage diminishes and all but erases the conjugal act as the consummation of the public verbal commitment sacramental act?

### Article 5:

What if Wojtyla's (later John Paul II) concept of the Theology of the Body has its roots in St. John of the Cross's personalism?

### Article 6:

What if sexual morality is a good example of the effect that the modernist and empiricist view of the body has in terms of understanding Catholic sexual morality?

### Article 7:

What if the human person is a body, rather than merely having a body?

### Article 8:

What if through the incarnation of Jesus, the Son of God, the Word became flesh and dwelt among us?

What if through God, the Son's assuming a human body, the body of all humans acquires an infinite value?

## Article 9:

What if original happiness, the beatifying the "beginning" of man (as related in Genesis), whom God created "Male" and "Female", the spousal meaning of the body in its original nakedness: all of this expresses rootedness in love?

## Article 10:

What if St. Paul's apostile's (letters) give evidence of an organic (natural, fundamental) link between purity and love?

## Article 11:

What if through His passion and death, Jesus Christ, restored man's hope of eternal life that was man's destiny from the beginning?

## Purpose Statement

This e-Book is meant to be a companion treatise to myself/understanding guide book What is Man? Male and Female. The five philosophers' views in What is Man? answer this question. The view that a person holds regarding human sexuality is directly derived from his or her, answer the question, What is Man? Male and Female. What does it mean to be human?

## Introduction

The view that a person holds regarding Human Sexuality is directly derived from his or her answer to the question, What is Man? Male and Female. What does it mean to be human?

This Mini E-Book Human Sexuality in John Paul II and Teilhard de Chardin is based on my interpretation of Pope John Paul II's view of Human Sexuality as he wrote it in his world acclaimed book <u>Man and Woman He Created Them – A Theology of the Body</u>, and on Teilhard's classic <u>The Phenomenon of Man</u>.

Both are theistic views based on philosophy, science and religion.

This mini E-Book is meant to be a companion treatise to my Self-Understanding Guidebook,

<u>What is Man? Male and Female</u>

Published on 11/11/2011 and launched on February 15, 2012.

## Article 1

## Human Sexuality – God's Unique Plan

"Then God said, Let the earth bring forth all kinds of living creatures: cattle, creeping things, and wild animals of all kinds."….

"Let us make man in our image, after our likeness. Let them have dominion over the fish of the sea, the birds of the air, and the cattle, and over all the wild animals and all the creatures that crawl on the ground.

God created man in his image; in the divine image he created him, male and female he created them." Gn. 1: 24, 26-27.

If we read the entire chapter we learn that in the beginning of time God created all things inanimate and animate. He simply summons them into existence. Genesis is not a scientific book so the mechanics of creation over and above God willing it are not to be found.

When it comes to the human being we come to the uniqueness of his plan.

"Let us make man in our own image, after our likeness."

Orthodox Christianity believes that God is a Trinity of three persons, Father, Son, and Holy Spirit, each distinct but also equal to each other. They are so united by divine love that they constitute One God, one Divine Being but three distinct persons. So, man made in the image and likeness of God is a person created for his own sake, not an animal created as a thing to be used by others.

In Chapter two of Genesis, verse seven is the second story of creation: "The Lord formed man out of the clay of the ground and blew into his nostrils the breath of life, and so man became a living being."

Thus man from the beginning was a living body, a living being, a body-spirit person. God then places the man in a beautiful garden to cultivate and care for it. Notice the "man" is alone and is not designated as "male".

Biblical scholars tell us that this second creation story is much older than the first one. It places the creation of man before the rest of the animate world.

Also the dialogue of love continues among the Trinity who desire to share this love with others and so the Lord God said, "It is not good for the man to be alone. I will make a suitable partner for him." He brings all the animals and birds for the man to see and name but none proved to be a suitable partner for the man. Gn. 2: 18, 20.

The man is cast into a deep sleep and while he's asleep God removes one of his ribs and closes up the place with flesh. He then builds this rib into a woman. Then he brings her to the man who said, "This one at last is bone of my bones and flesh of my flesh; this one shall be called 'woman,' for out of 'her man' this one has been taken. That is why a man leaves his father and mother and clings to his wife, and the two of them become one body. The man and his wife were both naked yet they felt no shame."

Man becomes male and female, two distinct persons, masculinity and femininity who know in their innocence the spousal meaning of the body. They know the selfless free giving of each person to the other in true love. Man is now constituted as fully made in the image and likeness of God who is love and light, compassionate and merciful.

God's unique plan for man at his very beginning of existence has come to be, but not for long! Gn. 2: 21-25.

## Article 2

## Uniqueness of the Human

The Human is unique among God's creation in that from a single Man God creates two persons, a male, what we now call man, and from the male's own body, a female, a woman, to be man's lifelong partner, of one flesh with him. "The two of them become one body." Gn. 2: 24.

In Matthew 19: 3-8 Jesus engages in a dialogue with the Pharisees who questioned him about the indissolubility of marriage based on Moses allowing a man to divorce his wife through "the promulgation of a divorce decree." Mt. 19: 7.

Jesus answers them "Because of your stubbornness Moses let you divorce your wives but at the beginning it was not that way. I now say to you, whoever divorces his wife…and marries another, commits adultery, and a man who marries a divorced woman commits adultery." Mt. 19: 9.

So the indissolubility of a valid marriage which was the case with Adam and Eve ("at the beginning") still holds for Jesus. It is one of the evils that enters human history because of the Fall – original sin, the eating from that infamous tree in the Garden of Eden.

But the human being, male and female remain the only creation of God who are persons made in God's own image and likeness. They are not objects or things. Man entered the world as a "living soul" a "unified being" brought to life by the breath of God. (*Theology of the Body in Simple Language*, p. 14.)

The human body is not like any other animal body. Only the human knows that he knows. He has the capacity for reflective thought – one more way he is made in the image of God. He carries out distinctive human activities like tilling the soil. A man's body reveals who he is: a mind-body-spirit complex creation, created for his own sake. He is capable through creation and grace of becoming a partner with God through the covenant made with Israel and later through Jesus' Redemption.

Adam is to enjoy the garden and eat from all but one tree. If he does, "you will surely die." Gn. 2: 16-17. "Die is a foreign term to Adam but he realizes that it is the total opposite to all that he has experienced in the Garden of Eden. He knows that he is entirely dependent on God for his very existence and for that existence, that life, to continue. He has a free choice between life and death, between death and immortality and he knows this from the beginning. (*Theology of the Body in Simple Language,* pp. 14-15.)

## Article 3

## Love in the Divine Plan

Human love in the Divine Plan begins with the creation of the first man as a solitary body-spirit, alone. God and Adam notice that it's not a good thing for man to be alone. Since Adam cannot find a suitable partner among all the animals as he is naming them – a helper – who could be so united to Adam as to be a part of him, God decided to remedy the situation by creating woman, Eve, whom Adam immediately accepts as a gift – the gift that he needs to be fully human. With the coming of Eve the first Man becomes a man (the first male) and Eve becomes the first woman (a female). Each of their bodies is so constructed as to complement the others – each is a gift that is both given to the other and received from the other freely and joyfully.

Among all living animal bodies, the human body is unique because through a free act of self-giving it expresses love in the image of God's love in which humans were made. The human body with its power to express love allows the persons to be a gift to each other as well as being a source of fruitfulness and procreation.

The heart of Christianity is self-giving love first exemplified in the life, passion, death and resurrection of Jesus Christ. This self-giving love is unique to the human person because while other creatures reproduce, they do so by instinct and don't love each other in the image of God's love because that is not how they were created.

Christian love grows in each Christian as he or she gives it away to others or in marriage to a special other. Created by the love of the love of the Trinity, a love God wished to share, humans are called to love each other in return and it is only by doing so that we discover who we are and why we are here on Earth.

Self-giving love, emptying one's self to serve others not only brings us the most happiness and fulfillment we can find in this life but it also prepares us for the complete fulfillment of seeing Love, The Light, and be filled to the overflowing with joy and happiness in the life to come. We were meant to be in complete communion with God and each other. God initially gives us his love when he infuses our unique spirit into the fertilized egg in our mother's womb and we become a human being. We spend a lifetime developing this gift of free and complete self-giving especially when a man and woman freely give their bodies as gifts of love to each other in the nuptial relationship.

## Article 4

## The Spousal Meaning of the Body

Our bodies, male and female reveal who we are scientifically and theologically. Science can examine our bodies physiologically in minute detail down to our sexuality, cells, and DNA. But that's it. Theologically our bodies reveal our innermost and unique personhood and they make our innermost being, the invisible (our soul) visible.

In Genesis 2:23, Adam's exclamation upon seeing Eve as "flesh from my flesh and bone from my bones" reveals how the masculinity (male) and femininity (woman) of the human body reveals man as a person, a being, that his very bodiliness is similar to, i.e. made in the image and likeness of God." This "body" reveals the "living soul" which man became when God breathed life into him.

In Genesis 1:27 which contains an account of the creation of the visible world, "has meaning only in relation to man.... man appears in creation as the one who has received the world as a gift....and the world has received man as a gift." (Theology of the Body, pp. 180-81)

The spousal meaning of the body refers to the fact that man (male and female) are persons willed for their own sake who cannot fully find themselves except through the free gift of self to each other in the conjugal act. This spousal meaning of the body also explains man's original happiness in his original innocence. (Theology of the Body, p. 189) This original innocence before the Fall of Man has to do with the rightness of intention in the exchange of the gift of themselves to each other. This exchange has to be a welcoming and accepting one in which each sees the other as a person not an object or thing to be manipulated or used by either partner. The exchange has to be reciprocal if the effects of "finding oneself" are to be revealed to each other and increase in each exchange. (Theology of the Body, pp. 195-197)

After Original Sin, The Fall, original innocence was lost and the achievement of the spousal meaning of the body "was to remain as a task given to man by the ethos of the gift" it would now really constitute a task, something to struggle to achieve rather than a given as it was in man's existence prior to the Fall. Human love was still meant to be a free gift of one person to the other but it became a more difficult task to keep the free gift of self always as one person to another person and never as a relationship to the other as an object to be used solely for one's own desire and pleasure. Shame entered the picture. Nakedness was no longer free of shame as in original innocence. Men and women began to cover their bodies, at least their genitals with clothing.

Although there are real differences in the state of man before the Fall and after it, man is still created in the image and likeness of God. Every new human being whose body is created by the conjugal love of his parents and who becomes human by the direct infusion of a soul created especially for that new human being by God himself is as fully human as were our first parents in their original innocence. Each of us is the result of the exercise of the spousal meaning of the body which is reflected in each of us. (Theology of the Body, pp. 213-214)

## Article 5

## John Paul II's The Theology of the Body

Wojtyla's (later John Paul II) concept of the Theology of the Body has its roots in St. John of the Cross's personalism. He adopts this view as his own and "focuses on the lived experiences of personal subjectivity…. Love is the gift of self; spousal love is the model gift of self that reflects the love that the persons of the Trinity, Father, Son and Holy Spirit have for each other." (Theology of the Body p.94) Among other modern concepts of personal subjectivity proposed by Descartes, Kant, Schilea and Schmitz state:

1. Matter is nothing more than the "without of things" – their physical structure – it is value free. It represents modern science's ambition and increasing power over nature. (Descartes)
2. Setting religion and morality on the foundation of the dignity of the individual person, the autonomy of the individual person is "the only true value to which everything else must be subordinated." (Kant)
3. "Human Consciousness" (choice) "sets the terms for reality itself" (Schelea and Schmitz). This view is very similar to Jean-Paul Sartre's existentialist view that each individual person's freedom to choose is the ultimate value. There is no universal standard beyond the individual person's choice or freedom to choose. (Theology of the Body p.95)

Wojtyla's response to these "modern" previews of personal subjectivity in addition to what has been stated in the first paragraph above, is that "to be a person is to stand in relation to a gift…to live as a body that offers a rich natural expression for a the gift of self in a spousal love." He rejects the modernist views previously stated as "an attack on the body" which "together with all matter is simply an object of power to be manipulated as the scientific – technological knowledge makes such manipulation possible."(Ibid.)

"The spousal mystery" (meaning of the body) "is the primary place at which this defense must take place because the highest meaning of the body is found there. The body is much more than mere matter. It is a spiritualized body, just as man's spirit is so closely united to the body that he can be described as an embodied spirit. The richest source of knowledge of the body is the word made flesh. Christ reveals man to himself through the revelation of the mystery of the Father and his love – the Trinitarian exemplar of the relationship between the Father, Son, and Holy Spirit – a relationship of infinite love." (Theology of the Body, p. 96 and 97) "The order of nature and the biological order must not be regarded as identical." These two orders can only be regarded as identical when the elements of these two orders are – "accessible to the methods of empirical and descriptive natural science." (Ibid) That is when the information being considered is subject to empirical verification in a laboratory following established rules of scientific method.

## Article 6

## The Empiricist's View of Human Sexuality
## Versus The View of Catholic Morality

Sexual morality is a good example of the effect that the modernist, empiricist view of the body has in terms of understanding Catholic sexual morality. For the modernist, the sexual urge is "only the sum of functions…directed toward a biological end…reproduction." For the Catholic Moralist, "the sexual urge owes its objective importance to its connection with the divine work of creation." (Theology of the Body, p. 98)

Where do these conflicting views of the body lead in terms of our sexuality example?

In Wojtyla's view the order of person and of nature are strictly united. In the order of love a man can remain true to the person only in so far as he is true to nature. If he does "violence to nature" he also "violates" the person by making it an object of enjoyment rather than of love.

In the modernist view, the empiricist view, the "biological order" as a product of the human intellect, has man for its immediate author so man has power over nature as his scientific – technological knowledge dictates. To this way of thinking, contraception and its mirror image, in vitro fertilization seems to be the most "natural things in the world." (Theology of the Body, pp. 98-99)

For the orthodox Bible believing Christian, the theology of the body which spells out the meaning and purpose of human sexuality begins in the first two books of Genesis, the creation stories of man, as male and female persons with spiritualized bodies that were meant to be free spousal gifts to each other.

While the Fall, called Original Sin, made it more difficult to achieve the spousal meaning of love, it did not remove it as the goal of human sexuality. Redemption was needed and promised. The promise was kept in Jesus.

For human living in the twenty-first century, the theology of the body is nothing but an extended commentary of this fundamental truth: Christ fully reveals man to himself through the revelation in his body of the mystery of divine love – the love that exists between the Father, Son, and Holy Spirit, three divine persons – a trinity who is one God.

This mystery of divine love is made visible through the gift of sexual difference, man as male and female and the call of the two to become one flesh – the male – female communion of persons – a sharing in the trinitarian communion through Christ's spousal relationship with the church. (Theology of the Body, xviii) The sacrament of Marriage is the essential public action and sign of the language of the body in its true spousal meaning.

The increasing phenomenon of couples living together before marriage diminishes and all but erases the conjugal act as the consummation of the sacramental act. Sexual intercourse in these unions is nothing but concupiscence of the flesh, not the conjugal act. The sign of the verbal commitment to each other before a priest, deacon, or minister and at least two official witnesses followed later by the consummation of the verbal commitment by sexual intercourse constitutes the full sacrament of marriage experiencing the language of the body and its spousal meaning in the free and complete self gift of each to the other as persons.

## Article 7

## The Value of the Body

"The human person is a body, rather than merely having a body….Man expresses himself in the body and in that sense is the body." (Index, p. 681, Body 1, Theology of the Body)

In this earth life, at least, man, the human, is an inseparable body-spirit complex. Every person consists of a "within" (every form of psychism including his or her individual soul which is directly created by God at the moment of conception) and a "without" (his or her body in its entirety – all its parts – but especially his or her brain and nervous system through which his "within" becomes observable in this earth life. The human body has an infinite value because the eternal Son of God, Jesus Christ, chose to be incarnated – to become fully human by being born of Mary as a human body with a fully human nature with the exception of Original Sin.

The core beliefs of who Jesus was and is, was first expressed in the Apostles' Creed which stemmed from St. Peter's teaching in the Church of Rome. This creed was made more explicit and detailed in the first two ecumenical councils of Nicea in 325 and 381 A.D.

Seventy years after the second council of Nicea, in 451 A.D. the fourth ecumenical council at Chalcedon defined Christ still further… "one and the same Son, our Lord Jesus Christ: the same perfect in divinity and perfect in humanity, the same truly God and truly man, composed of rational soul and body; consubstantial (of one substance) with the Father as to his divinity and consubstantial with us as to his humanity; like us in all things but sin." (Catechism, p. 118, par. 467)

A little over one hundred years later in 553 A.D., the fifth Council of Constantinople had to clarify further about Jesus "there is but one hypostasis (person) which is our Lord Jesus Christ, one of the Trinity." (Catechism, p. 118, par. 468) These solemn teachings sealed the view of the infinite value of the human body because the Son of God chose to assume a human body and nature – to be incarnated.

In his helpful guidebook, Theology of the Body in Simple Language, Sam Torode writes that "By upholding human dignity Jesus words about lust affirm the value of the human body. The body shares in our dignity as persons, just as much as the spirit." (Sam Torode, p. 94)

St. Paul in 1 Corinthians, Chapter 3, verses 16-17 reminds us of what our body really is. "Are you not aware that you are the temple of God, that the Spirit of God dwells in you?  If anyone

destroys God's temple, God will destroy him. For the temple of God is holy, and you are that temple."

It is through our body that we perceive the spirit for we are embodied spirits. The body, its physical appearance, our facial expressions like smiling, frowning; our speech, i.e. what we say and how we say it, etc., expresses the person. As strange as it may seem in our sex saturated culture, the bodily sexual embrace between a man and a woman in the committed relationship of marriage expresses both an invisible and visible love, a full giving of each to the other that is both physical and spiritual reality. The exercise of this <u>person</u> to <u>person</u> (<u>not</u> object to object) relationship is a form of prayer as well as a reflection of how a man and a woman image the Trinitarian relationship of the three Divine Persons with each other.

It is true that the human being is often sinful (commits adultery in his or her heart by looking upon even one's wife or husband <u>lustfully</u>, thus reducing the other person from being a person, a <u>subject</u>, to being an <u>object</u>. But that doesn't mean that the body is evil. It simply means that humans are capable of misusing their bodies. Habitual indulgence in lustful behavior, in thought or action, clouds our vision until we are no longer able to perceive the original meaning of the body. Rooting out lustful behavior, especially if it has become habitual (like immersing ourselves in pornography) is not an easy task. In fact it is an impossible task if we think we can change such behavior on our own. We have to first admit that we are powerless to do so and then that we have to lean on the grace of God to help us root out our sinful desires regarding the meaning and use of the sexual aspects of our bodies.

It is very true that it is far easier to <u>acquire</u> a bad habit than it is to change it. Perseverance in prayer, repentance, and avoiding the "triggers" that lead to lustful desire and behavior, are the way and this way involves following Christ to Calvary.

Our conversion journey is lifelong. It involves joy and sorrow, perseverance, and a <u>willingness</u> to walk the way of the cross especially with regard to treating our own bodies and those of others as temples of the Holy Spirit. But the reward of eternal life (and peace of mind and heart in this life) – Easter resurrection when our glorified body will be reunited with our soul – a fully human life forever, is well worth the journey.

## Article 8

## The Human Heart

Through the incarnation of Jesus, the Son of God, The Word became flesh and dwelt among us. Through God, the Son's assuming a human body, the body of all humans acquires an infinite value. Sin is a matter of the human heart being dominated by one or more of the following three forms of lust:

1. "the will to power" (Nietzsche). The Apostle John calls it "the pride of life."
2. "the desire to acquire and protect wealth (Marx). The Apostle John calls it "the lust of the eyes"
3. "the sex urge" (Freud). Jesus condemns the "lust of the flesh" but this term does not equal "the sex urge" as such, but rather the way this urge is allowed to exist in our innermost selves, and the way our sex urge thoughts manifest themselves in our bodily actions (Sam Torode, p. 94)

The first lust "the will to power" or "the pride of life" is found throughout history in the numerous men and some women for whom the lust for power led them to be the most cruel of dictators, and in the Roman Empire to be divinized – to be gods. In the twentieth century persons like Mao in China, Adolph Hitler in Germany, and Joseph Stalin in Russia were "Gods" in their countries with their followers the Communists and Nazis obeying these men's every dictum. The result was horrible carnage, World War II, Concentration Camps, The Holocaust and unimaginable evil.

In the twenty-first century Radical Islam is driven by lust for power by force over others because their interpretation of Islam leads them to the use of force to convert the "infidels".

The second lust "the desire to acquire and protect wealth" (Marx) and "the lust of the eyes" can also be found throughout human history.

In ancient Greek and Roman History for example, the desire for conquest of other nations was often driven by the desire to possess the particular wealth of another nation(s) like precious metals and stones, spices, cloth (silk), etc.

In our own day the acquisition of fossil fuels like oil are the driving force behind much of our diplomacy and foreign policy often disguised under more noble sounding motives. The desire to acquire and protect wealth is at the heart of corruption in many governments including our own. There is nothing immoral about working honestly and being successful in a business or other adventure – wealth in itself is not an evil – it all depends how the wealth is acquired and how it is used.

The third lust, "the sex urge" (Freud) and "the lust of the flesh" are the concepts of Passion (eros in Greek), romantic love, and modern day eros (erotic or the sexual attraction) that draws a man and woman to unite their bodies, are common ways of understanding the word "erotic".

Although the Bible doesn't use the term "eros", eros is present in Genesis in the Call by God to Adam and Eve to become united in one flesh. So, eros is at the foundation of the communion of persons. The Bible uses the term "ethos" (morality, ethics) to mean "the condition of the heart with regard to what is true and good." (Sam Torode, p. 97)

"When romantic love is channeled to this end, it is deeply connected to ethos, namely what is good and right in God's eyes." (Ibid., p. 97)

When "eros" is defined as striving for selfless love – to give all of one's self – all of one's love – all of one's body to the other – to make them happy , joyful, fulfilled, and when this same attitude and behavior are held by one's partner we achieve the spousal meaning of the body – a true nuptial union. Mutual pleasure between two persons is one of the beautiful and good things of a mutual self-giving love. A person cannot achieve such self-giving love if he or she is habitually lustful – looking upon his or her partner as an object to be used for self-gratification. We must examine not only bodily behavior but also our innermost thoughts and deepest impulses because it is from these that our behavior comes. There is nothing spontaneous, free, or lasting about lust of the flesh. It doesn't aspire to goodness, truth, or beauty.

All Christian morality finds its fulfillment in self-giving love. We are called to be free so we can serve one another in love. (Ibid., pp. 100-112)

# Article 9

## Reconnecting Body and Heart

"Original happiness, the beatifying 'beginning' of man (as related in Genesis), whom God created 'Male and Female', the spousal meaning of the body in its original nakedness: all of this expresses rootedness in love." (Theology of the Body, p. 190, 16:1)

Love is rooted in the innermost depths of the human heart. When this self-sacrificing, total mutual self-giving takes place between two spouses, a man and a woman, in their sexual union, romantic love is deeply connected to what is good and right in God's eyes. The heart and body are reconnected "by reconnecting body and heart", the "without" (exterior) of man with the "within" (the interior, heart, soul, spirit). "Christ introduces a new morality (ethos), a new way of living as an embodied (body – soul) person." (S. Torode, p. 102) Constant self-examination of our hearts is a necessity to see whether our innermost thoughts and actions are directed toward redemption of the body – toward guarding our hearts and controlling our impulses.

This cannot be done without an intimate and ongoing personal prayer relationship with Jesus Christ in which we both speak and listen. It is a relationship in which Wisdom Himself points out to us the persons, places, and things we must avoid that build lust of all three kinds in our hearts.

We must be willing to persevere through temptation that is enhanced by the images we see embedded in the Media and on the streets.

Self mastery is a life-long process. If we have grown accustomed to giving into our impulses, this weakness must be balanced by frequent and sincere Confession. The grace of Reconciliation gives us forgiveness, wipes the slate clean – we have fallen, repented of it, and risen again. But our impulses bring images into our inner most thoughts the longer and more frequently we have given into them. These images, easy to acquire continue to haunt us back to the slavery that giving in to our sinful impulses brings with it.

As we persevere and are willing to suffer, we "will begin to experience the body as a gift" (Torode, p. 103) – as the temple of the Holy Spirit – a gift that has been ransomed for us by the passion and death of Christ.

Freedom will come gradually. It is the result of persevering in self-control and it is the foundation of love between persons.

We will grow in purity of heart which will make it possible for us to act with self-giving, self-sacrificing, total love between ourselves and our spouses. Our bodies and hearts will grow in their connectedness.

True purity must begin in the heart for the heart is the dwelling place of our innermost thoughts and values. These values are the source from which our bodily actions spring.

Our conversion journey must see a continuous growth in our "Living by the Spirit." We can not do this on our own and the good news is that we don't have to! Our strength to grow in living in the Spirit is the power of Christ operating within us through the Holy Spirit. "God has poured out his love into our hearts by the Holy Spirit, whom He has given us." (Rom. 5:5) (Sam Torode, pp. 104-08)

Freedom in the Spirit is made possible by the Transforming power of Christ's redemption. As Teilhard de Chardin writes in his book, The Phenomenon of Man, Christ's redemption begins with the human, man, who is the leading shoot of evolution, but it is not limited to man. Christ saves the entire universe. He is part of Omega (God). It was through His Word (Christ) and for His Word that God, the Father created the entire universe. So, Christ is an indispensable part in the evolutionary process. All evolution before Christ was a preparation for His coming. All development since His coming is simply the completion of His Mystical Body. Christ provides the basic elements of hope and love. Hope is essential to progress, the will to "keep going", and love is essential to convergence (humankind coming together) and unity. Christ is the love object who will draw all men together. ( B.J. Fleury, What is Man?...p. 67)

Without this Love (Christ) dwelling in the innermost thoughts and values of our hearts we cannot escape the bondage of sin or gain freedom of spirit that will enable us to learn purity of heart.

If Purity of Heart is absent, the reconnecting of Body and Heart is impossible.

## Article 10

## Purity and Love

St. Paul's Epistles (Letters) give evidence of an organic (natural, fundamental) link between purity and love.

At the surface level, purity equals abstaining from immortality. At a deeper level, purity equals an experience of love inscribed by God on the whole human person. So, honoring the dignity of the whole human person is to reverence the image of God in the body. (S. Torode, p. 119)

The word "love" as Jesus and Paul used it is defined as selfless giving, self-sacrificing, focusing on the "other" rather than on myself. It is the kind of love Jesus demonstrated for us in his earth life from his birth in a manger, his thirty years spent as Joseph, the carpenter's son, helping his father and then supporting his mother as a carpenter.

Jesus spent his final three years of earth life as a wandering rabbi with no place to lay his head, continually giving of himself in teaching, healing, surrendering himself to the tortures of His passion, dying a criminal's death by crucifixion – all for our well being and redemption.

Reverence for the image of God in our bodies is stressed over and over in St. Paul's letters. Among his many such passages is the following one which I meditate on often, "Are you not aware that you are the temple of God, that the Spirit of God dwells in you? If anyone destroys God's temple, God will destroy him. For the temple of God is Holy, and you are that Temple." (1 Cor. 3:16-17)

How can one fail to reverence his body seeing that since the body is the temple of God, and that the Spirit of God, the Holy Spirit, the Spirit of Love dwells there – and that Purity is an experience of this Love?

Purity and Love are so intimately united that you cannot have Love in God's sense of the word and not have Purity. Nor can you experience purity without love!

Purity, trust, and openness between persons are essential if we are to engage in a communion of persons as in the martial union. (S Torode, p. 119) By creating man in the image of God, precisely as male and female, God inscribed His love in the human body. Our complementary bodies, masculine and feminine, carry the sign of the gift. The physical construction of male and female bodies, are obviously complementary to each other through natural physical union. They are meant for each other.

Purity is experienced by abstaining from lust in thought and deed and by appreciating the dignity of the human body given by Christ assuming such a body for himself and then coming by His grace to dwell in each human body that welcomes Him. Because our body bears the sign of a gift, we are called to fulfill that sign by actually becoming a gift to ourselves and others. (S. Torode, p. 122) How do we accomplish this task?

We accept and live by a view of man as a body-soul integrated and complex being.

The view that we accept that defines man, the human, shapes our own self-image, the way we parent our children, the way we treat others, the education we advocate, and the therapeutic strategies we would use in the helping profession.

Art, for example, in any of its forms such as written, painted, sculptured, photograph, film, can either encourage or destroy purity of heart.

What happens when the body, especially the nude body, becomes subject of art in any of the forms listed?

The question is not whether the body should be described, but rather how it is described. Classical Greek sculpture of their heroes, the statue of David, etc., are examples of the body depicted with dignity.

Bodies depicted in such a way encourage lust in the viewer such as images of sexual activities that are solo or between persons of the same or opposite sexes.

Is the body (bodies) engaged in sexual acts art or pornography? The problem is reducing the human body to an object of lust, instead of reverencing it as a subject, a sign of a person.

In pornography, art becomes a lie. The body created as a fee gift of male and female spouses to each other in marriage is perverted – depersonalized – reduced to an object of lust – enticing the viewer to engage in the same behavior. We oppose pornography out of respect for the dignity of the body of the performer and the viewer not out of any puritanical or "body is evil" point of view.

If one adopts the so called "naturalism" in art view whereby a person demands the right to reproduce everything that is human including pornography, are realistic depiction of humanity, then the body is indeed reduced to an object for lustful pleasure rather than the full truth that man as created in the image of God, a person, and not an object must be considered. (S. Torode, p.128)

There are far too many examples of addiction to pornography that results in destroyed lives, destroyed marriages, cruelty of all kinds, the degradation of both men and women as persons, subjects, and of physical and spiritual death to allow any thinking persons, and especially any Christians from advocating, participating in, or tolerating, pornography. If we want to be truly free in the Spirit, to be persons who put love of God and Neighbor up front in their lives, we must acknowledge the essential link between purity and love. By so doing, and living out this love we can get a foretaste of heaven on this earth, peace, and some measure of contentment; and eternal peace and joy when we finally reach our destiny of eternal life with God.

## Article 11

## Resurrection Destiny – The Perfection of Human Bodiliness

Through his passion and death, Jesus Christ restored man's hope of eternal life that was man's destiny from the beginning.

At death our lives are changed, not ended. Our soul (spirit), lives on in either Heaven, Hell, or temporarily in Purgatory, but our bodies decay. The human being as a body-soul complex temporarily ends. We are not fully human again until the resurrection of our bodies at the second coming of Jesus.

At the resurrection when the body and soul are reunited, marriage will cease to exist because our bodies participate in a completely new state of life where the purposes of the earthly marital union to image the Trinitarian relationship and procreation, cease to exist. We regain our glorified bodies in the fullness of the image and likeness of God. (S. Torode, p. 139)

We remain masculine and feminine individual persons for eternity. Resurrection restores life to each person with a perfect integration of body and soul. The opposition between body and soul that we experience in earth life will come to an end. Concupiscence is over. Even though our bodies as well as our souls (already spiritual in earth life) will be spiritualized and divinized (filled with God's own life) we will not be any less human but more.

We will reach a fullness of life permeated by the Divine that even the holiest of the holy earth humans could never possess.

Through Divinization we do not become God but we enter into a new state – humanity, body and soul in perfect union with God – "intimately connected to the Trinity in a perfect union with God and in a perfect communion of persons without losing our individuality as persons". (S. Torode, pp. 141-42)

In Christianity, unlike Buddhism or Hinduism, the individual body – soul integrated complex of each person is a permanent feature which has a beginning at our conception but thereafter is immortal. Our souls do not become part of some all embracing spirit that swallows up our individuality. The nuptial meaning of our bodies in earth life in which espouses experience the full self-giving of each other in marriage gives way to what Christ teaches. Our destiny is for a body-soul intimate full communion with him.  In eternal life, God will gift himself to each of us in the most personal way. As the scripture tells us, we will see him as he is, "We will rediscover in a new dimension the same nuptial meaning of the body" – "the ultimate meaning of our sexual embodiment (man, woman) "in a virgin" (non sexual urge) "union with God." (S. Torode p. 143)

This union with God embodies the "sight" (on intimate experience) of Holy Trinity, the most perfect communion of the three Divine Persons. Such an unbelievable gift from God has to draw us to give ourselves completely to him.

In Heaven our attention will be riveted on God. In focusing on Him we will also see as in a mirror the entire cosmos anew in Him. We will also know our fellow humans, friends and family and even ourselves within the infinite life of the Trinity. Thus we will experience what we have confessed over and over in our creed, "I believe in the communion of Saints." As we have noted, I am me forever, an individual person but also in the relationship of a perfect communion of persons. The communion that the resurrection brings is the final realization of the "nuptial meaning of the body and the perfect realization of God's Trinitarian love in the hearts of men." (S. Torode pp. 144-45)

Our glorified bodies will still be signs of our personhood, the way we communicate with others, and the means by which we show expressions of selfless love.

Our God is a God of the living – the living Christ who was raised from the dead by his Father. It proclaims God's victory over death for "The last enemy to be destroyed is death." (1 Cor. 15:26)

The resurrection of Christ points to the destiny of humans, and to the end of history, when Jesus will hand back to the Father everything that the Father created through and for his Son.

## Summary

### Article 1:
"Then God said, Let the earth bring forth all kinds of living creatures: cattle, creeping things, and wild animals of all kinds"….

"Let us make man in our image, after our likeness. Let them have dominion over the fish of the sea, the birds of the air, and the cattle, and over all the wild animals and all the creatures that crawl on the ground.

God created man in his image; in the divine image he created him, male and female he created them." Gn. 1: 24, 26-27.

### Article 2:
The human is unique among God's creation, in that from a single Man, God creates two persons, a male, what we now call man and from the male's own body, a female, a woman, to be man's life long partner, of one flesh with him. "The two of them become one body." Gn. 2: 24.

### Article 3:
Human Love in the Divine plan begins with the creation of the first mans a solitary body, spirit, alone. God and Adam notice that it's not a good thing for a man to be alone. Since Adam cannot find a suitable partner among all the animals as he is naming them-a helper-who could be so united to Adams to be a part of him. God decided to remedy the situation by creating a woman, Eve, whom Adam immediately accepts as a gift-the gift that he needs to be fully human. With the coming of Eve the first Man becomes a man (the first male) and Eve becomes a woman (the first female). Each of their bodies is so constructed as to complement the others-each is a gift that is both given to the other and received from the other freely and joyfully.

### Article 4:
Our bodies, male and female reveal who we are scientifically and theologically. Science can examine our bodies physiologically in minute detail down to our sexuality, cells, and DNA. But that's it. Theologically our bodies reveal our inner most and unique personhood and they make our inner most being, the invisible (our soul) visible.

### Article 5:
Wojtyla's (later John Paul II) concept of the theology of the body has its roots in St. John of the Cross's personalism. He adopts this view as his own and "focuses on the lived experiences of

personal subjectivity....love is the gift of self: spousal love is the model gift of self that reflects the love that the persons of the Trinity, Father, Son, Holy Spirit have for each other.

## Article 6:
Sexual morality is a good example of the effect that the modernist, empiricist view of the body has in terms of understanding Catholic sexual morality. For the modernist, the sexual urge is "only the sum of functions...directly toward a biological end...reproduction." For the Catholic Moralist, "the sexual urge owes its objective importance to its connection with the divine work of creation." (Theology of the Body p. 98).

## Article 7:
"The human person is a body rather than merely having a body....Man expresses himself in the body and in that sense is the body." (Index, p. 681, Body 1, Theology of the Body). In this earth life, at least man , the human, is an inseparable body-spirit complex.

## Article 8:
Through the incarnation of Jesus, the Son of God, the Word became flesh and dwelt among us. Through God, the son's assuming a human body the body of all humans acquires an infinite value. Sin is a matter of the human heart being dominated by one or more of the following three forms of lust:

1. "the will to power" (Nietzsche). The apostle John calls it, "the pride of life."

2. "the desire to acquire and protect wealth" (Marx). The apostle John calls it, "the lust of the eyes."

3. "the sex urge" (Freud). Jesus condemns the "lust of the flesh" but this term does not equal "the sex urge" as such, but rather the way this urge is allowed to exist in our inner most selves, and the way our sex urge thoughts manifest themselves in our bodily actions. (Sam Torde, p. 94).

## Article 9:
"Original happiness, the beatifying 'beginning' of man (as related in Genesis), whom God created 'male and female', the spousal meaning of the body and its original nakedness: all of this expresses rootedness in love." (Theology of the Body, p. 190 16: 1).

## Article 10:
St. Paul's apostiles (letters) give evidence of an organic (natural) fundamental link between purity and love.

At the surface level, purity equals obstaining from immorality. At a deeper level, purity equals an experience of love inscribed by God on the whole human person. So, honoring the diginity of the whole human person is to reverence the image of God in the body (S. Torode, p. 119).

## Article 11:
Through his passion and death, Jesus Christ restored man's hope of eternal life that was man's destiny from the beginning.

At death our lives are changed not ended. Our soul (spirit), lives on in either heaven, hell, or temporarily in purgatory, but our bodies decay. The human being as a body-soul complex temporarily ends. We are not fully human again until the resurrection of our bodies at the second coming of Jesus.

# Bibliography

1. <u>Catechism of the Catholic Church</u>. English translation, United States Catholic Conference, Liguori, Mo., Liguori Publications, 1994.

2. Deacon Bernard J. Fleury, Ed.D. Sixty years of preparing couples for marriage, processing many difficult annulments, participation in Marriage Encounter and fifty-six years as a husband, father and grandfather.

3. Deacon Bernard J. Fleury, Ed. D. <u>What is Man? Male and Female</u>, Create Space 2016.

4. Dr. Richard A. Spinello. "The Rehabilitation of Charity," <u>Homiletic and Pastoral Review</u>. Ignatius Press, 1348 10th Avenue, San Francisco, Ca., Volume CXI, No. 5, February, 2011.

5. John Paul II. <u>Man and Woman He Created Them, A Theology of the Body</u>. Translation, Introduction, and Index by Michael Waldstein. Boston, Mass., St. Paul's Avenue, 2006.

6. St. Joseph Edition of <u>The New American Bible</u>. The Confraternity of Christian Doctrine, Washington, D.C., 1970. Author uses this edition for endnotes in text.

7. <u>Revised Standard Version </u>most frequently used by English Translators and at times <u>The New American Bible </u>which differ at many points from the version used by John Paul II, namely, the official translation published by the Conference of Italian Bishops (CEI). Eg. of differences is Mt.5:28 RSV: "Everyone who looks at a woman <u>lustfully </u>has already committed adultery with her in his heart." CEI version: "Whoever looks at a woman <u>to desire her</u> instead of <u>lustfully</u> 21 times but uses <u>lustfully</u> 343 times.

    a. "In order to avoid difficulties of this sort, the English Scripture quotes have been conformed to the CEI translation, always with an eye on the original Greek or Hebrew."

8. Torode, Sam. <u>Pope John Paul II's Theology of the Body in Simple Language</u>. Lexington, KY, Philokalia Books, 2008.

www.ingramcontent.com/pod-product-compliance
Lightning Source LLC
Chambersburg PA
CBHW071321280526
45788CB00004B/1973